THE ART OF THE NAP

DOW P. WINSCOTT

THE ART OF THE NAP

Cover by
Christine Winscott

Illustrations
Mike Bills

Editor
Editor Mike Valentino

SPECIAL ACKNOWLEDGEMENTS

Diane Curtis
above all others, for patiently enduring my
endless prattle concerning The Art of The Nap

Scott M. Smith
for always keeping a straight face when I discussed The Art of The Nap

Christine Winscott
for making The Art of The Nap look just like a real book

Joseph Schwartz
for making me feel like I might actually be an author

Bridget Hindert
for her always gentle and convincing encouragement

Leah Roach
for her unquestioning enthusiasm and spot-on feedback

Dr. Gerald Lofthouse, M.D.
for keeping me both well and reasonably calm

Richard Marten, Police Commissioner
for his early support and confidence building ability

THE ART OF THE NAP

Foreword

A few years ago I called my great pal John Muno who was spending a week at the home of a mutual friend in sunny Arizona, just to see how he was doing. Our mutual friend, like John, is a very successful businessman who enjoys sharing his millionaire's life and could write his own book on how to successfully mix business with pleasure. From past experience, I knew that John's week would have been filled with long lazy days lolling around his host's expansive pool, occasional trips to a nearby mountain lake to tool around in his exotic powerboat, and of course, a bit of nightlife as well. When I asked John how his week was going he responded enthusiastically, "Just great! I've already had three naps!" Now, if you are not a napper or, if you are lucky enough to be able to nap anytime you wish, you might be surprised at John's response and maybe even a little disbelieving. But, if you are a true napper who only infrequently gets to nap, you understand his enthusiasm perfectly. Hey, pools and partying are wonderful additions to anyone's schedule, but a nap – now that's Heaven!

George Bernard Shaw (how's that for adding a bit of class to a foreword?) once famously stated, "There are two kinds of people in the world – the kind that think there are two kinds of people and the kind that don't." With less cleverness, but plenty of sincerity, I propose that when it comes to naps there are also two kinds of people in the world: the kind who view them narrowly, as a monumental waste of time, nothing more than the indulgence of disengaged slackers or classically lazy people. And the other kind - those enlightened souls who embrace naps as a blissful means to achieving inner peace, restored energy, and, occasionally, even enlightenment. The Art of The Nap is not intended to convert those who hold naps in disdain, but to assist and validate those who have already achieved some measure of success in folding them into their lifestyle. But if you are a napping naysayer, please read on with an open mind and if you deign to join the ranks of napping devotees, know that you will be warmly welcomed. And even if you don't join us, you will certainly find yourself with a better understanding of the "other kind of people."

CHAPTER ONE

A (very) Brief History

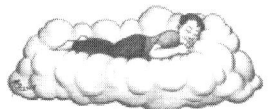 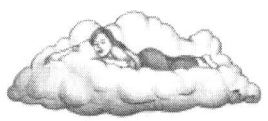

You know, you could easily skip this chapter. Honestly, if you are very busy, maybe feeling the urge to nap, or just want to skip ahead to a more meaty chapter, fine. Go right ahead. This really is just a more or less obligatory chapter in a book like The Art of The Nap.

Somehow we seem to have reached the point that for a subject to be taken seriously, it must have a history. A historical perspective seems to make almost any subject a little more important and, in some odd way, more legitimate. And napping, possibly more than any other common human behavior, suffers from an undeserved lack of both legitimacy and respect. Lets face it, if you are anywhere south of the age of about five, talking about your nap is almost certain to raise the questioning eyebrow of anyone within easy earshot – this despite the fact that those with the mildly disapproving look on their faces may have enjoyed a delicious nap themselves just hours ago. Ah guilt! Sigmund Freud coined a term for this behavior while developing his theory of psychodynamics – he called it projection; sort of cleansing ourselves of guilt by assigning a personal attribute to others; *"Napping? Good Heavens no! I can't believe anyone would waste even a moment of their life by napping."* Yeah, right. And by the way, is that a pillow wrinkle I see on your cheek?

Freud was actually being kind. Such a divergence between expressed attitude and deed might also rightfully be called hypocrisy. But that's maybe a tad bit harsh, so I won't go there. In any case, read on if you wish, but no guilt if you bail out of this historical perspective. Don't worry, there's not going to be a test on it later!

How about the cradle of civilization as a starting point for our brief history? Or at least one of the cradles. Civilization, it seems, was more of a nursery than an only child situation. Which is actually probably a good thing, or the world it's turned into would probably be pretty boring today. Anyway, if you were to learn that archeologists had discovered ancient glyphs in a very early Egyptian tomb that clearly depicted Pharaohs enjoying naps, what difference would it make to you? Sure, there may be some measure of satisfaction knowing that these regal and powerful leaders passed at least some of their time in the exact fashion you do (I refer to napping, of course, not slaying those that have devoted their lives to building your final resting place). And it might help to explain how those people spent their time when they weren't busy developing the most perplexing written language ever or contriving lethal plots against various factions of their own families. It's also possible that they dreamed up some or all of this while taking naps, of course, but we don't have sufficient evidence at this time to say for sure. And anyway, this is a celebration of the benefits of napping, not a brooding contemplation of a darker side.

But this sort of musing only steers us away from the history (yawn) of napping. My initial effort to gain insight into the napping habits of early Egyptians (really nothing more than a quick telephone call to the Chicago Museum of Natural History) didn't get me very far. After several unanswered telephone transfers, I found myself back at the receptionist's desk. I asked her what she thought about the napping habits of early Egyptians, but she politely declined to comment. With a limited amount of time available for historical research and an even more limited interest, I turned to the Internet (which the ancient Egyptians never had, with good reason – imagine URL's in hieroglyphics) and discovered that all contemporary nappers are in good historical company. Very good historical company. Consider these nappers -

My sentimental favorite has to be Thomas Edison. Like so many other educators, my seventh grade teacher, Mr. Phillips, tried valiantly to captivate his students with stories of historical figures whose efforts had shaped their lives. Frankly, until he got around to telling us about Edison's unconventional practice of taking several short naps each day, I was unimpressed. As a side note, I should point out that Einstein must not have been much of a napper or surely my teacher would have mentioned it. Yet, his wild hairdo does make it seem quite plausible that he had a bad case of bed head, maybe from frequent naps, unless he woke up that way and never touched it with a brush all day long. OK, back to Mr. Phillips. With his help, I was able to conjure the picture of Edison working maniacally on his inventions and then periodically dropping onto a small mattress in his laboratory and falling fast asleep only to awaken a short time later and get back to inventing. Could it be that his inspiration came to him while sawing some Z's? To me it was fascinating. Even now, when I discuss napping with folks, the story of Edison and his serial napping behavior frequently emerges; Mr. Phillips apparently wasn't the only teacher that used Edison's naps to help his students appreciate science. I doubt that he gave it much thought, but certainly Edison could have added "power napping" to his long and illustrious list

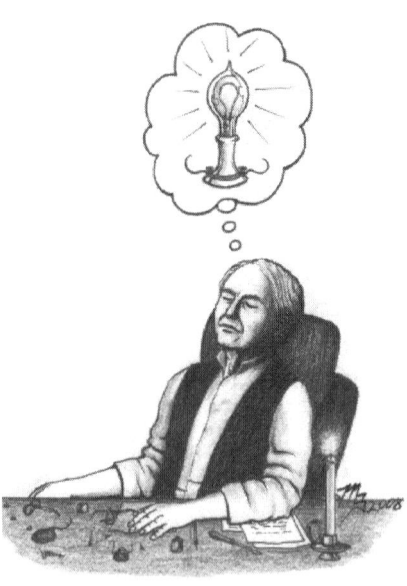

of inventions. I can only imagine the confusion, though, when he applied for a patent for it. Millions of others would have come forward claiming that they had been doing the same thing for years, and would want a share of any profits derived from this new concept. Edison chose to be content with the electric light bulb and a few hundred other novel innovations.

In my research I also discovered that napping played a major role in Presidential history as well. President Bill Clinton is just one in a long list of White House nappers that includes Ronald Reagan, John F. Kennedy, and Lyndon Baines Johnson to name a few. President Clinton took his naps in the afternoon and it is reported that he left instructions that he be disturbed only for the most urgent business. I'm not sure what would constitute *unimportant* business for a president, but fortunately I was not one of the aides that had to make the disturb/don't disturb decision. I am not certain just where in the White House President Clinton did his napping, but I like to imagine many were taken in the familiar Oval Office, with the President tipped back in his office chair. A beautiful picture. Snoring may or may not have been part of the scene, but I doubt anyone would bring it to his attention.

Not all historical nappers were men. Eleanor Roosevelt gave luncheon speeches all over the country, providing the White House with important citizen reaction to national policy even as it was being developed. By all accounts Roosevelt was a very gracious and persuasive speaker and the luncheon speeches she gave certainly impacted American history in ways still not fully understood. Despite her success in speaking to the American public, however, Roosevelt nearly always felt anxious at the thought of addressing her luncheon crowds. Her solution? A brief nap an hour or so before speech time. She reported that the naps left her calm and ready to confidently face her audiences. Hard to ask more than that of a nap, wouldn't you say?

Add a few more to your list of famous and historic nappers – Leonardo Da Vinci, John D. Rockefeller, Napoleon Bonaparte, even Gene Autry (sorry, no mention of Trigger's napping practices). What do these historic figures share in common besides being nappers? Each and every one of them is noted not only for their specific skills or talents, but also for the sheer volume of work they generated. It becomes clear that any small amount of productivity we might seem to lose while napping can be gained back exponentially as a result of the nap.

So the history of napping is, as you can clearly see, one that is long and quite glorious. As we move forward into a deeper exploration of our intriguing topic, you can rightfully be proud to be a part of this wonderful tradition. Your personal journey into napping may still be in its early stages, but who knows what your contribution may be to its illustrious history?

CHAPTER TWO

You Call That A Nap?

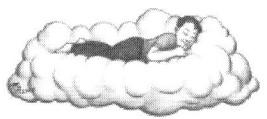 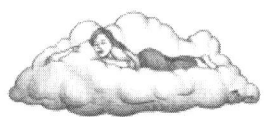

Maybe we haven't all done the following, but most of us have been dangerously close to it or have our own, personal version. You're on the sixteenth straight hour of a twenty-one hour road trip to Florida, or California, or…well, you get the picture. Despite umpteen cups of coffee, the radio blaring and a 70 mile an hour blast of air screaming through the open side window - *you are falling asleep.* Your eyelids seem as heavy as manhole covers as you fight to keep them from squeezing shut. You give it your best, most valiant effort, but they close for seconds at a time before something snaps you wide awake – usually the blare of someone else's horn or the bumpy ride that precedes running completely off the road. Since you are reading this now, there is a pretty good chance that you parlayed extraordinary good luck with some desperately needed good sense and pulled over. Either that or the docs at the ER did an exceptionally superb job keeping you alive!

But let's keep it positive and assume that, once refreshed, you were able to proceed safely on your way. What exactly was it that occurred during those brief yet potentially fateful moments when your eyelids were closed and your mind drifted from the highway to blissful dreamland? You need to understand that what happened was not a "nap" in the proper sense of the word. Oh, sure, your body was screaming out with fatigue, but "drifting off" while at the wheel is actually a case of simply losing consciousness from sleep deprivation. Definitely not a nap, or even anything resembling a nap.

Let me propose another scary scenario. You're sitting in the back of your classroom during a sterling lecture delivered by your favorite professor or maybe sitting around a board table, attending a critical corporate staff meeting. Your notebook is open, your pen is poised, you are trying for that earnest, "I'm totally with the program" look on your face and - *you are falling asleep.* You fight it, but your eyelids slowly droop as the lecture becomes a drone in your ears. For a moment your mind flashes back to that awful time you almost crashed your car...and it actually seems more pleasant than this! You are jerked back to wakefulness by the weight of your head lolling sharply forward or backward. Yikes! It hurts like hell and you feel certain that you have permanently damaged your spine and have been "busted" to boot. Still, as you sweep the room with sidelong glances it appears, to your great relief, that no one has noticed your brief departure from the land of the awake and the alert. On the other hand, maybe everyone did see you and they're holding back their snickering to not embarrass you. Studying their faces, you just can't be sure. Are they polite or just oblivious? It's tough to tell.

So what happens next? You guessed it – you repeat the whole hideous process again. This time you are certain that you have been noticed and you are right. Nothing says, "I am dis-involved" quite as eloquently as falling asleep in a room full of people who are wide-awake. You can only imagine how everybody's opinion of you has just plummeted like a rock. All because of a few seconds of catching some unintentional and unplanned Z's.

While neither of these examples describes a nap, both

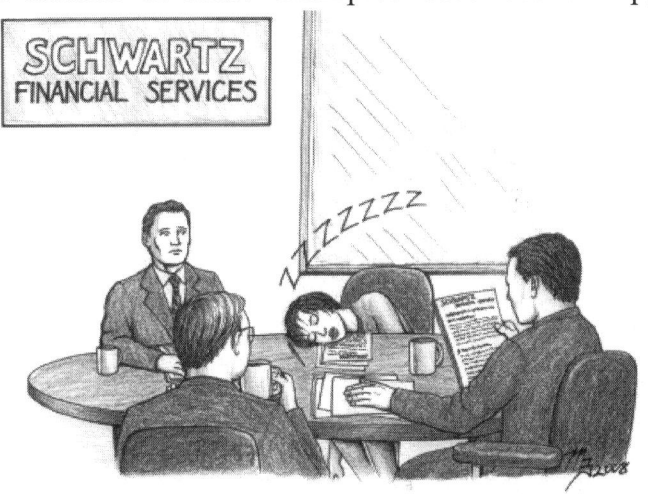

provide ample evidence of how effective and possibly even critical a nap -- the genuine sort -- might be to your success (to say nothing of your survival) in life. And though there is a rich assortment of nap types and napping strategies available to all of us (oh yes, many different types of naps are out there just waiting for our enjoyment), these two frightening scenarios illustrate a common denominator of all naps: *choice.*

Choosing to take a nap, contrasted to falling asleep by

accident, is like the difference between joining the Army and getting drafted. True naps are completely voluntary. Your nap is exclusively yours to choose to enjoy now, choose to postpone until a later moment, or to restructure in a multitude of fashions to meet your specific need. So, if the sleep you are getting is not enough to fully fuel your wakefulness, a preemptive nap can literally save the day. Now is the time for all good men and women to seize the power of when, where and how to nap!

As you will soon discover, there are numerous styles of naps and napping, and we will be taking a close look at several of them. For now, consider this – *we fall asleep, we take naps.* Whoever first strung those particular words together was quite wise indeed.

CHAPTER THREE

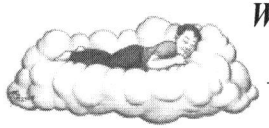

Where? When? How Long?
Those Are The Questions

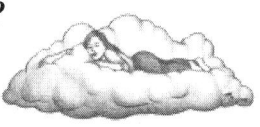

Well, we have established that careening down the interstate in a sleep deprived state or the horror of falling asleep at the corporate meeting, does not lead to what most of us would call a nap. A disaster? Oh yeah, most assuredly. Humiliating and career denting, yep, for sure. But again, certainly not a nap. This being acknowledged, let's take a look at some of the component elements of a successful napping experience. Like an elegant soufflé, it involves a thoughtful mixture of ingredients.

What does napping have in common with the real estate market? Location, location, location. No question about it, your choice of location to enjoy your next nap is going to play a crucial role in it being a positive experience rather than a disaster. Some folks head straight to their bedroom when the urge to nap begins its irresistible tugging. Others prefer the comfort of their favorite couch or easy chair. These two time-honored napping locations aside, the fact of the matter is simple – there is no absolutely right or wrong place to nap – the choice is all yours. It's a big world out there, so why limit yourself to only two possibilities?

Let's face it, not all choices are created equal, and some decisions that we make are clearly superior to others.

Nonetheless, sometimes the conflict between the logical limitations of an available napping location and the nearly overwhelming urge to nap finds us nudged into a less than great decision. In a perfect world, the best place to nap is wherever we happened to be when we chose to take a nap. OK, but what about those of us (I'm pretty sure this includes everybody this side of Valhalla) who don't live in a perfect world? We may have some tough napping location decisions ahead of us – but that's not necessarily a bad thing. You can turn this seemingly difficult situation into something positive. In fact, you may be quite surprised by how many choices you really have or can create.

The key is to use your imagination. The world is chock full of potential spots for you to nap. If it's safe (and legal) you may even want to find an outdoors location for your slumbering. There really is no limit to the possibilities, if only you follow the urgings of the creative napper that dwells within all of us.

Second only to location is the question of just when to nap.

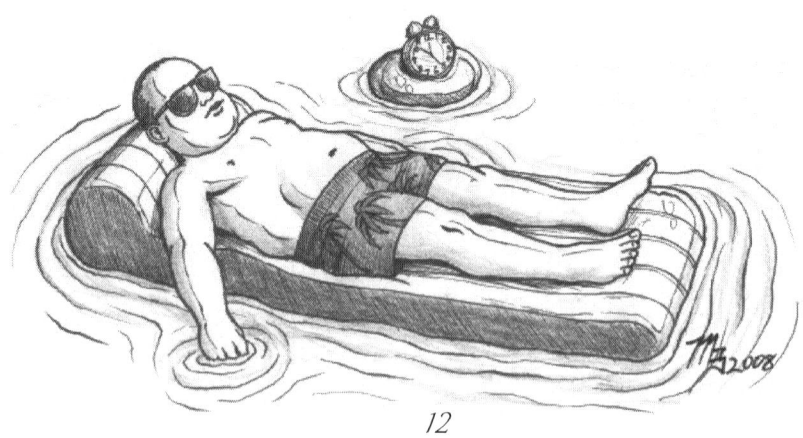

Some napping purists I know insist that the very notion of pre-planned napping is nearly anti-social and that only the spontaneous nap is truly virtuous and full of joy. Other nappers stoutly maintain that a scheduled regimen of napping is precisely what elevates their productivity, nourishes their emotional well being and just plain suits their lifestyle. Who's to argue with either of these positions, so vehemently defended by their adherents? Both meet individual preferences and predilections and their diversity is nothing more than a reflection of just how freeing the whole concept of napping can be. Still, each of these positions begs its own set of consideration and we will explore them just a little further on.

This last consideration is a little trickier. You'll see what I mean. *Just how long is a nap, anyway?* Even the word itself, nap, has that abbreviated air about it that evokes a sense of brevity. But just how brief? It seems reasonable that a nap be considerably shorter than our nocturnal sleep period. But again, how much shorter? I told you this was tricky. We could, of course, simply confer the same mantle of individuality to the length issue that we have to location and timing. But that seems like the easy way out. My compromise position (you are welcome to establish your own) on the length of a nap vacillates between finite, concrete periods of time – say as little as five minutes at a minimum to around an hour and a half maximum.

We can add to that a criterion that is a whole lot softer - *nap until you have gained what you needed or wanted to gain from your nap.* This last model may leave those of you who have had the experience of oversleeping a little uneasy. Flashbacks of that nearly heart stopping feeling, as you realized you would be late for work, maybe had missed a crucial appointment, or had somehow fumbled an important responsibility keep us as one with our alarm clocks. Oddly, it seems that "over napping" almost never occurs. It may be that when we nap, we manage to stay close enough to full consciousness that our internal alarm clock is more effective. Clearly, this is an issue that warrants further scientific investigation, and we will delve into the latest research findings to help you come to your own personal sense of nap length. In any case, for our purposes here we will soon be looking at ways to keep you anxiety free as you pursue and enjoy your delicious nap.

But under any circumstances, always keep this in mind: a nap, whether desperately needed or simply much desired, is *still a nap – a joyful pleasure only you can give yourself and something to be richly savored.*

CHAPTER FOUR

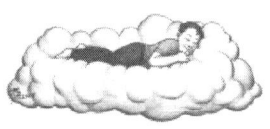

A Little Science
Goes A Long Ways

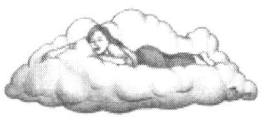

There is a good reason why the title of this book is The Art of The Nap, not The Science of The Nap. The science of sleep is a very young, but vigorous discipline and has shed a great deal of light on what occurs when we slip into the nether world of nocturnal sleep and the role that sleep plays in our lives. Sleep scientists have clearly established that sleep plays a critical role in the maintenance of our physical, emotional and even mental health. A number of enlightening references related to sleep science findings have been included in the citations section of this book. Consider them a bonus as they relate more directly to traditional, nocturnal sleep than to naps, but be sure to check them out; it will be time well spent.

This book, however, is dedicated to the celebration of naps and those who take them and has almost nothing to do with science. Naps are not just the little brothers or sisters of nocturnal sleep; they have very different features in terms of both our physiological responses and social reactions to them. And they require their own brand of, "care and feeding". The focus here is on helping you gain the greatest benefit possible from your naps based on personal observations, experiences of others and deep contemplation on naps and the lucky people who get to enjoy them. Those of you who are reading this right now know who you are. All that being said, it is time to take a little departure from the path of the art and dip our napper toes ever so gingerly into the world of science. I know, I know. You're holding a book with the word Art in fairly large letters on the cover and now, with no real warning, you find yourself about to come face to face with what some of my more elitist academic colleagues call "real" science. Trust me. Not only will I make sure that these next few paragraphs are completely painless for you, I give my solemn word as a fellow napper that the information will actually be of some use to you in the pursuit of perfect napping. And for all we know some of the most ardent nappers out there may well be research scientists. After all, napping seems to refresh the brain, so perhaps that's the secret to what keeps those folks so smart. It's a fascinating thought, isn't it?

In any case, for starters, you may be a little surprised to learn that there really is no definitive explanation for why we sleep. Sure, it would be easy enough to just say that we fall asleep because we get tired. And that explanation almost works until we take into consideration that sometimes we get tired (sleepy?) but don't fall asleep. Maybe we are just having too darn much fun to give in to sleepiness and shrug it off, or maybe we are faced with a crisis that demands our full conscious attention for an extended period of time. You may have noticed yourself, that if you stay awake just a couple hours or so beyond your normal bedtime, falling asleep often becomes difficult, if not downright impossible. It's almost as if there is a sleep bus and if we aren't there to meet it at our normal stop – it rolls off without us. And sometimes the next sleep bus is a long time coming!

There are many theories concerning human physiology and how it relates to sleep, but the fallback explanation revealed through research is exquisite in its simplicity. Sleep is restorative; *we sleep to recharge our physical, emotional and mental batteries.* Personal support for this somewhat simplistic theory can be found in the fact that when we are more active than usual or are under a greater than usual level of stress, we usually respond by needing more than our usual length of sleep. But that's where we usually run into trouble because needing, unfortunately, is not synonymous with getting.

While there is disagreement and even some confusion among sleep researchers as to why we sleep, there is nearly universal agreement concerning the effects that sleep deprivation has on human functioning. Consider how you perform after a poor night's sleep, or worse yet, without any sleep at all. Chances are pretty good that the next day you are cranky (a rather polite term, wouldn't you agree?), much less productive than usual, and prone to make poor decisions. Plus, you probably felt tired and... well, sleepy. For many of us the differential between how much sleep we need and how much we actually get is more than just a little problem. Lack of sleep has a powerful effect on our cognitive processing abilities and has been directly linked to many major disasters. A modest but telling list of these sleep deprivation related disasters is chronicled in the citation section of the Art of the Nap. Take a look if you need any reinforcement of the idea that sleep is a good (read *essential*) thing. The alternative is downright scary.

The amount of sleep each of us needs each night varies widely between individuals and, as noted, often is related directly to what happens to be going on in our lives at any given moment. But the trend, overall, definitely has not been in the right direction. Sleep researchers have discovered that, on average, Americans get approximately one hour less sleep every day than they did 100 years ago. So much for the labor-saving devices of our modern world, huh? Yet, most of us know of someone who claims five hours a night is plenty, a startling concept to those of us who have trouble dragging out of bed after eight or more hours. This problem is especially significant with teenagers and with older people. Recent research reveals that adolescents may actually require as much as ten hours of sleep each night to support their normal developmental process while many elderly people meet their sleep requirement by taking serial naps throughout the day and have a more abbreviated stretch of uninterrupted sleep during the night. With all of the individual variations considered, eight hours of sleep each evening, on average, seems to be the figure reported by the majority of those surveyed. But again, this is the amount of sleep that the average person feels is right for them, not necessarily the amount they get each evening. It's the same as with eating. We all know how many calories we ought to have every day – but not all of us stick to a well-balanced diet as strictly as we should.

Consider this for a moment. We have established that while there are a number of possible explanations for *why* we sleep, scientific research has established that we *need* sleep to recharge our selves in order to deal effectively with the challenges of the next day. If we don't get enough sleep, our overall performance will likely suffer (to say nothing of those unfortunate enough to be around us after our abbreviated sleep) and the result can range from a minor annoyance to an outright disaster. Now, add this to the mix. Nearly all sleep researchers report that fully twenty percent of the adult population suffers from insomnia at one time or another. Twenty percent – that's astounding! We all know that insomnia refers to an inability to sleep, but it isn't that simple. Sleep researchers have isolated three distinctly different manifestations of insomnia; failure to fall asleep, failure to stay asleep, and early awakening. The subject of insomnia has long been the butt of jokes and has often been central to comedic sketches, but (like hemorrhoids) it is no joke to those who suffer from it.

The net result of any of the forms of insomnia is…that's right, a reduction in how much time we spend asleep. Those suffering from insomnia generally get some sleep each night, but not nearly the amount that they really need. In other words, they have not been fully restored. The good (make that *great*) news is that there are remedies and treatments for insomnia that range from behavioral therapy to medically supervised programs. The bad news is that a great number of people who suffer from insomnia simply choose to live with the problem. And again, because the sleep they routinely get is below the fully restorative level, these folks are subject to a variety of deficits in their day to day lives.

So now comes the $64,000 question. Would a nap help? It would seem so, but there are many considerations that must be made. As wonderful as a nap is and can be, it is probably not the long term solution to a serious sleep disorder. If your night time sleep is frequently interrupted or consistently leaves you feeling less than restored and unprepared to meet the your daily challenges, my strong encouragement is for you to consult with your health caregiver and discuss possible causes and remedies. Again, the citation section of The Art of the Nap provides many useful resources.

OK, that's it for the science section of this book. Don't worry, there won't be a quiz later...but you will get extra credit if you take a nice, relaxing nap. As the old ad slogan said, *"better living through science (and napping!)"*.

CHAPTER FIVE

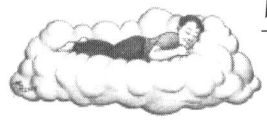
Where, Oh Where to Nap?
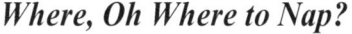
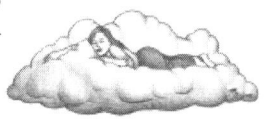

Life would be simpler if we could just plop down wherever we happened to be when we felt a nap coming on. Simple maybe, but it would sure make for a crazy landscape. Just imagine picking your way over all the slumbering bodies in your workplace, shopping spots and other frequented areas. Inevitably, you'd trip over some poor soul and wake them up. Not to mention how noisy it would be with all of that snoring. No, selecting where you take your naps requires some forethought to optimize their quality.

"Safety first" should be your motto when scouting out possible napping locations. Let's face it, when you nap you are increasing your vulnerability. It's a little disturbing to acknowledge that such a joyfully pleasant experience requires safety considerations, but better safe than sorry. Ultimately, taking the right precautions will enhance the overall experience and the pleasure will be increased. Do you feel safer when you click your car seat belt into place? Of course you do. And once you have taken that simple safety measure you can be off and on your way, enjoying your drive. When it comes to naps, there are many simple measures that can be taken to assure your safety while you are off in Napland.

What is a safe location for napping? Home nappers don't even think about safety when they lay down to sleep in the comfort and privacy of their own dwelling place. Whether curled up on their bed or stretched out on a comfy couch, they doze off without a care in the world, surrendering themselves to their luxurious and restorative nap experience. It's with good reason that from time immemorial people have said that there's no place like home. You could easily paraphrase that to *"There is no place like home to take a nap"*.

But what about on the job naps? It pretty much depends on your work situation. If you're a police officer, for example, dozing off in your cruiser probably isn't a good idea and will most likely lead to some pretty stiff discipline. The same goes for airline pilots (even when your 747 is lumbering over the middle of the Atlantic on auto-pilot, napping is still not recommended for those in charge of the cockpit). On the other hand, those who enjoy the sanctuary of a private office are in a great position to nap safely. An office chair securely positioned against rolling and your head resting against the wall (bring your own pillow!) may be a long way from a bed, but still makes an excellent improvised napping nest. Or you could even take it one step further. While the idea may seem a little bold to you, I know of one ambitious napper who invested in a very ingenious collapsible cot that she stores in a corner of her office, always ready to be pressed into service.

The corporate movement towards a world of cubicles rather than fully private work spaces is in full bloom and is not likely to reverse itself. Many cubicle dwellers may be unnecessarily discouraged from an at work nap. Again, a strategically placed chair (careful with those wheels!) and your head against the cushy (usually) cubicle wall and you are off to your brief slumber. The key here is communication. Letting your supervisor know that you wish to substitute a few minutes of "shut eye" for your regular break period is a good start. To help overcome any resistance that may be encountered, you might want to pass along an article that highlights the work benefits associated with napping – not difficult to find. If you get the "green light," make sure that your cubicle neighbors know your napping schedule to avoid unnecessary interruptions.

Sadly, only a very few of us are fortunate enough to work for organizations sufficiently enlightened to provide "napping rooms" for their employees. These blessed souls typically

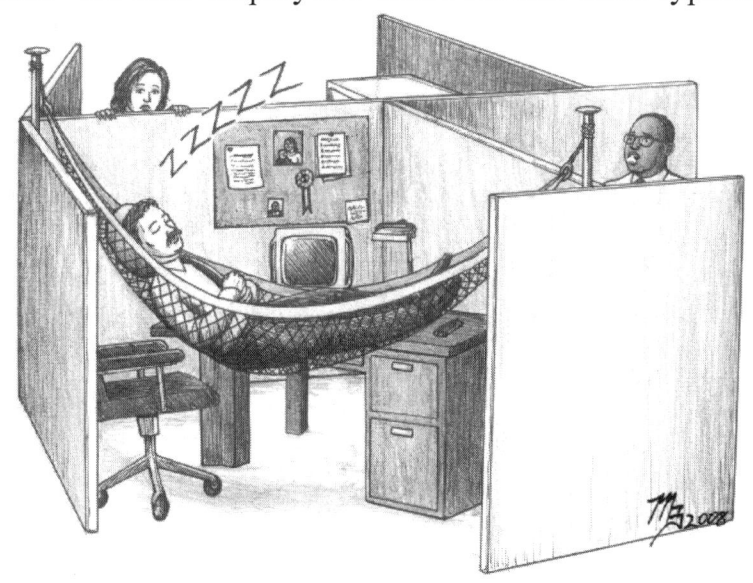

are able to trade off their traditional 15 or 20 minute work breaks for a chance to stretch out and take a short nap. The wise employers who provide this little perk are not just nice people who are sympathetic towards nappers, they are savvy folks who understand that a quick nap is restorative in ways that a typical "coffee break" simply is not. Rested and relaxed workers are more productive and less likely to be involved in work place accidents. Though their number is growing, "nap friendly" companies are still rare and so few that it would be a mistake to even imagine that a groundswell trend is in motion. But, as the true benefits of napping become more widely understood, we may see one take life. And keep this in mind – if you are ever in the corporate position to move your organization in the direction of being nap friendly, you could become a legend in your industry. Really.

The rest of us have to be more creative in selecting our safe napping spots. Taking a nap in a more public place requires judgment. Good judgment. Classrooms, for college students, can make excellent napping spots. Pick a classroom that is being actively used, but is temporarily empty between classes. Usually you will have from 15 to 30 minutes from the time one class is dismissed and the next class begins. Grab a chair at the rear of the classroom, get as comfortable as you can and lean your head back against the wall and drift off. The noise generated by students filling the classroom will generally be sufficient to wake you before the next class actually begins. Here's a tip: Drape a small digital music player around your neck and stick some ear buds in your ears; you won't be seen as a napper, just someone listening to their tunes and deep in reverie. Your brief nap concluded leaves you refreshed and ready to deal with your world.

I will have to avoid my many wonderful and esteemed librarian friends for this, but libraries make really excellent napping spots. First of all, most of them still subscribe

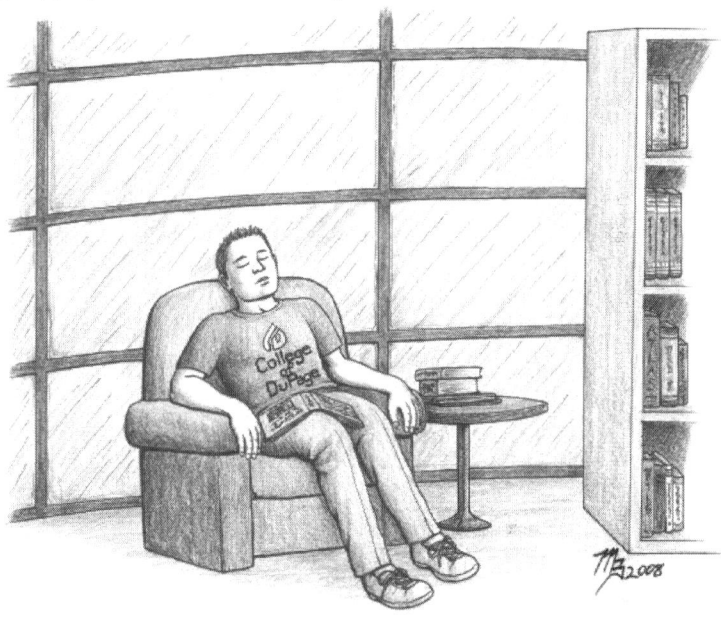

to the notion that their domain be relatively quiet. Good news for sound sensitive nappers. More good news – most self respecting libraries have very comfortable chairs strategically placed among the stalls of books. These chairs practically beg nappers to sink into their comfort and drift off for a few minutes. Another tip. Have a book on your lap or on the arm of the chair during your nap; you will be seen by all as someone who is just taking a moment's break from a good read. There is a double benefit to this, too, because if you have difficulty drifting off, a really boring book should easily do the trick.

Another candidate as a napping locale, because they are so often in close proximity to our workplace, is our cars. It's a tempting possibility, but you need to exercise some real caution. First of all, never ever take a nap in a car that is running. Never. No matter how new or how well maintained your car is, the possibility of a carbon monoxide leak is always a real threat. You don't want to turn a brief nap into something permanent! Next, if you do decide to nap in your car, keep the doors locked. All of them and always. If you are parked in a patrolled lot, let the patrolling officer know where you are going to be and that you are going to get a little "shut eye." Public safety folks typically respond very favorably to proactive requests for assistance, even if it is keeping a napper safe.

Many of us use public transportation on a daily basis. When a good novel, book on tape, or the Daily Bugle start to get a little stale, a nap might just fill the bill. Plus, the rocking motion of a commuter train or bus can be oh so conducive to napping. At both the beginning and end of our work day a little nap can go a long way towards refreshing us either for the work at hand or for whatever is awaiting us at home. You have instincts and you need to use them. If someone or something in the crowd on the train leaves you a little uneasy, take a pass on the nap and keep yourself alert – there will be other days for your commuter nap. Surprisingly though, public napping provides its own sort of safety net – your fellow travelers. It may seem slightly counter intuitive that public napping in a group setting is safe, but generally when people find themselves in trouble they are alone, not in groups. Even groups of near strangers.

Some people just love the great outdoors. And not all of these folks are hikers, sports persons, hunters or birdwatchers. Many are nappers. You see them everywhere. Some have their chins resting on their chests as they relax on a park bench. Others spread a blanket on the grass in the park and let the Sun's warming rays drift them into their napping bliss. Some are so dedicated to napping outdoors that they can even be seen bundled up against the cold of winter (generally with their faces positioned towards the Sun!) as they enjoy their outdoor nap. Now those are dedicated nappers! The outdoors seems like a pretty safe place to nap as long as you are around other people and not too close to the wildlife that rightfully calls the outdoors their home.

Clearly, being safe is the most important part of your napping location. But it isn't everything. Your location should be one that matches your own special requirements. Is it quiet enough for you? Is it near where you need to be before and after your nap? Are you going to draw unwanted attention?

Spend some time scouting potential napping sites as you move through your daily or weekly routine and watch for those that fill your bill. In no time you should be able to develop your personal portfolio of places from which you can successfully launch or sink into your personal nap land.

CHAPTER SIX

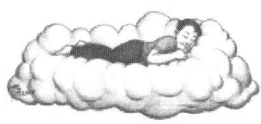

Napping Accouterments

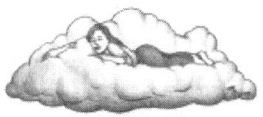

If, up to this point, you have been happily living your napping life without anything more than a pillow and maybe the occasional blanket, the concept of a nap benefiting from a few accouterments may seem puzzling or perhaps even downright laughable. After all, isn't one of the key joys of a nap the sheer simplicity of the experience? You find a comfy and safe place, close your eyes and drift off, awaking a short time later refreshed, relaxed, and rejuvenated. Accouterments! It probably reminds you of all of the time you'd need to spend getting yourself dressed for some kind of important, formal meeting or event. Doesn't sound very comfortable at all, you're undoubtedly saying. Who needs any accouterments? Well, actually *you* do. At least some of the time.

The accouterments of napping, unlike the accouterments of fashion, serve far more than a sartorial purpose. And that purpose is singular in its focus – to make your napping experience the very best it can be. Curious now? Read on.

When we consider the perfect length of a nap, it becomes clear that it is linked to both our need and the amount of time that we have available. For instance, our personal experience may indicate that we really require a one hour nap to gain the full restorative benefit needed. Big problem, though. Because of real life constraints, we have only thirty minutes available for our nap. What to do? Shrug off the idea of a thirty minute nap and just plug along, fatigued and under-performing? Or go ahead and take our nap, acknowledging that something is better than nothing and praying that we wake up in thirty minutes and not one hour? It's true-nothing is more "nap killing" than anxiety. If you have only ten minutes, thirty minutes or whatever minutes available to nap, you need the confidence of knowing, with certainty, that you will awake on-time. Without that confidence it will be more difficult to drift off and your nap will suffer from your tension. Well, you could carry a spare alarm clock around with you. Of course even the smaller ones are a little unwieldy and let's face it – they are ALARM clocks. Your intent is to assure you are awaken on time, not that all those around you be alerted that your nap is over.

Technology can be very useful for solving this problem. There is about a 100% chance that your cell phone has a built-in timer or alarm feature. If you can figure out how to set it (or you have a computer geek friend who can do it for you), you are in business. A great alternative is a wrist watch with an alarm feature. Not so many years ago only high end chronograph type watches included an alarm feature. Now you can find them for less than ten dollars in discount department stores everywhere. With only a few minutes of focused perseverance (and the assistance of the aforementioned geek or any child over the age of about 10) you can learn how to quickly set one to the time you need. The alarm tone itself? Anything from Take Me Out To The Ball Game to a more traditional alarm ring – but whatever you choose, you will be the one who is awakened without drawing undue attention from those around you.

I remember the first time I saw a Do Not Disturb sign. This simple but powerfully unequivocal message was hanging from a doorknob at a hotel I was visiting with my parents. Even at my tender age, this sign made a much larger and longer lasting impression than did the opulent hotel lobby and mirrored elevator. To think that something as simple as a three word sign could protect one from all the possible intrusions of life was nearly staggering (please remember, I was quite young). Now, a cultural phenomena related to technology has swept the world and has put nappers in the position of having their personal Do Not Disturb sign that they can take with them wherever they go. The phenomena I am referring to is the near epidemic use of personal music systems. You see them being used (worn, actually) everywhere – on public transportation, in the workplace, just about everywhere. Draped around the neck, with the little earbud speakers tucked into the ears of the user, these devices say Do Not Disturb with more eloquence than words could ever express. I think the psychology of this phenomena is linked to a slightly perverted version of the, *"It is not polite to interrupt when someone is in the middle of a conversation,"* maxim. Clearly, there is no real conversation going on, but we do have a sense that a communication, *some* kind of communication, is taking place when we see someone with the ubiquitous music device and the earbuds in place. Our response? Usually it is to move on, leave the person to themselves and maybe approach them later when the earbuds have been removed. We tend to put ourselves in the other person's shoes. If we were right in the middle of listening to a really great song, would we want somebody interrupting us? Of course not!

Accordingly, what could be more perfect for the napper who wants to be left alone to enjoy their nap undisturbed? You really only need the earbuds as they seem to be the most powerful of the visual cues. When the wires disappear underneath your shirt or jacket, people will just naturally assume that they are connected to an electronic acoustic device. Big bonus: Some of us actually like to fall asleep to

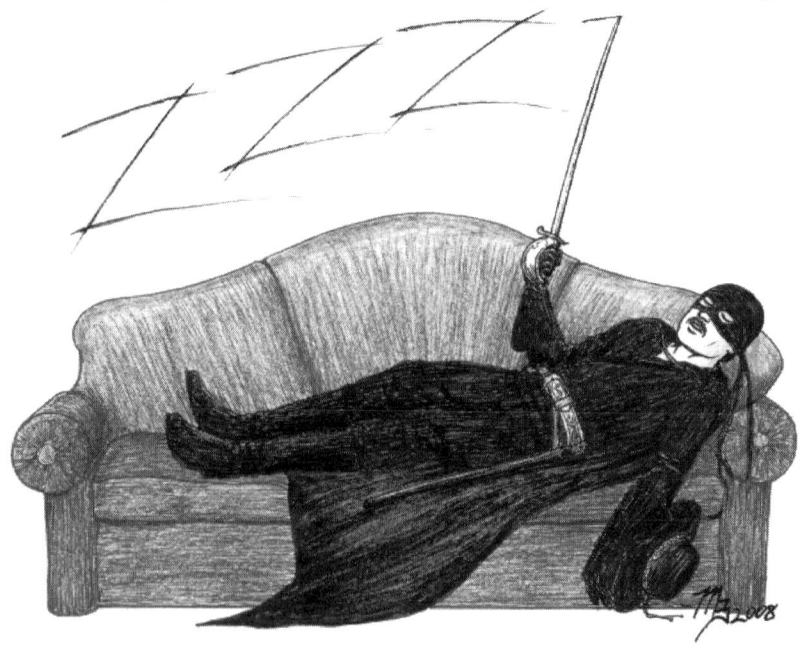

music, so if you want to, go ahead and dial up your favorite sounds to waft you into your nap.

For light-sensitive nappers, an easy fix is a sleep mask. First, think of Zorro, the dashing master swordsman of television fame, who made a cape, a horse and a sword symbolic of rescue from oppression. Now, imagine Zorro's mask in myriad brilliant colors and patterns and, of course, sans the cut outs he used to see beyond his mask. My guess is that Señor Zorro, as dapper as he was with his cape and sword, would have been mortified to be seen in anything other than his classic black mask. But don't feel bound by his tradition. Times have changes and it's OK for us to change with them. Today these masks can be found in a dazzling selection of colors and patterns in pharmacies, department stores and even health stores. For the very best selection and pricing you will probably want to head to the computer and shop on-line. Be prepared to be amazed at the choices available to you and the very modest pricing of this very useful napping accouterment.

When you were an infant and later a toddler, you most likely had your very own blanket. In fact, it may have been your very first possession. Usually it was a gift from an adoring grandmother or a loving auntie. Often these blankets were gender colored; blue for the boys and pink for the girls, of course. And even though many of us were fortunate enough to have more than one blanket, there was usually one blanket that became our soul mate. It, above all others, provided comfort when we were scared and boosted our confidence when we were uncertain. Ahh...our blankie. Even as an adult you likely have some trace memory of your blankie. What a sad day it was when we finally had to give it up and face the world on our own. Remember Linus for the Peanuts comic strip? He continued to carry his beloved blanket around with him far past the infant stage, deep into his childhood and (though we have no solid proof of this) most likely well into his teenage years.

Now, I am not advocating that you develop some quirky adult blanket dependency, but I am suggesting that you might want to select one for the exclusive use of your naps. When we sleep, our body temperature drops (sorry, little science here). Not radically, but often enough to wake us up. Have you ever taken a nap and awakened a little shivery? Yep, that's the sleep temp drop. Now don't confuse a napping blanket for that extra blanket you have stashed in the linen closet. No, a napping blanket needs to be lightweight, quite small, and easily folded into a very small package. You really only need enough blanket to cover the upper half of your body; just below the chin to around your waist level will keep you warm and comfortable. I know one person who keeps her napping blanket, sleep mask, wrist watch alarm, and portable music device in a soft lunch bag. Takes it to work with her every day just on the chance that she may take a nap. Very handy. No word where she keeps her lunch, though. Even if she has to spend a few dollars on fast food, however, it's well worth the sacrifice.

Finally, what good's a blanket without a pillow? I wish I had a clever answer to this would be riddle, but I don't. What I do have is a little advice. Skip the traditional shaped pillows and look for one of the many variations of neck pillows on the market. Travelers favor these crescent shaped pillows for the same reasons that many nappers do; they are small, comfortable, and unobtrusive. If, like my friend who packs her napping accouterments in a soft lunch bag, space is an issue, you might want to try one of the inflatable varieties. A few puffs and your once flat pillow is plumped and ready for napping duty. If you choose to purchase a neck pillow, make sure to get one that has a fabric-like cover; the vinyl variety heat up quickly when in contact with skin and become uncomfortable very quickly.

You and your personal napping habits will indicate what napping accouterments are most appropriate. If you can nap in your work office, don't bother with the sleep mask – go straight to the light switch. If a napping blanket is going to attract unwanted attention, ditch it. The bottom line is to take whatever steps might be necessary to assure success as you undertake this vital and rewarding endeavor. Always remember – *your nap is your nap, to be savored, treasured and if you choose, adorned with just the right accouterments.*

CHAPTER SEVEN

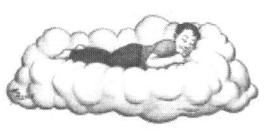

How Long
Is Your Nap, Anyway?

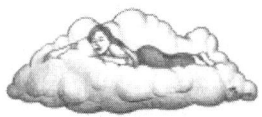

For most of us naps are such a delicious experience that we just can't seem to quite fathom the notion that there may be an optimum length for each of them. After all, don't all good things have their limits? Do you like ice cream? Would you really want to eat two gallons at a sitting? Of course not. How about your favorite pizza pie? Same thing. OK, maybe you could polish off a 16 incher all by yourself, but how about two of them (with all those heavy toppings) at one sitting? I doubt it. You would probably be better off skipping the ice cream or the pizza altogether rather than overdoing it to those extremes. And in much the same fashion, for each of us, there is an ideal nap length that not only satisfies our physical need for a "recharge," but also the more ephemeral requirements of what can be best described as our emotional equilibrium. Finding that optimal length of time for our naps is an exquisitely personal process that takes…well, time.

Here's a good question to ask yourself as you ponder how long your naps should be. *"How long would you nap if you were able to blissfully drift off only to awaken naturally, at your own body's bidding?"* Would it be fifteen minutes? Maybe an hour? Possibly as long as a couple of hours? The answer, of course, is that the length of your nap hinges on a multitude of factors. How much sleep you got the night before and the quality of that sleep will go into the nap length equation. The kind of day you are having and your expectations for the night or day that is still before you will certainly be a factor. And, without a doubt, just how much time do you actually have available for your nap? Yes, it really comes down to a whole bunch of *"it all depends."*

But let's take this out of the realm of theory and into the real world of napping. Let's face it, most of us don't often have the luxury of napping 'till we awaken "au natural." Our lives are just too busy these days, and we can't afford that kind of luxury. Realistically, our own self-imposed schedules as well as the schedules of others are going to strongly influence the length of most of our naps. You can't nap for as long as you want when the kids have soccer practice or you have an important meeting to attend. Life doesn't wait around for us to wake up – though so often it's fun to imagine a world in which it did.

At the end of Chapter One it was noted that we *fall* asleep, but that we *take* naps. I hope you haven't forgotten that important distinction. It's not just a clever play on words, rather, it's an inherent part of the nature of napping. Let me explain. You see, napping presents us with far more choices than does our normal nocturnal sleep. We get to pick the time, the location and to some extent, schedule the length of our naps. The choice is yours to make! You don't just "fall" into a nap. You deliberately set out to "take" a nap, as surely as you would take a walk, take a drive or even take on the world. It's an action verb, utterly devoid of passivity. You control it, and you should take full advantage of that control. Be sure to carefully select the location and timing of your naps, as well as their duration. These critical factors will heavily influence how satisfying you find your napping, and how much benefit they provide for both your physical and mental well-being.

"Power napping" is a term that has come into popular parlance over the past few years. The notion of a "power nap" is that it is fairly brief; typically just fifteen minutes or so, and primarily serves the purpose of on-the-job rejuvenation. Power naps may be the healthy, 21st century version of workplace coffee breaks. Of course, that's not to say that the time-honored and broadly practiced tradition of the coffee break is going to disappear anytime soon. Even in the face of their clear ineffectiveness, old habits (not to mention addictions to such things as caffeine) die hard. Yet it's clear that a major change is afoot, and why not? Everything else in our working lives has undergone serious transformations. So think of this as just one more way to leave behind the old world of coffee, cigarettes and poor health that once characterized most office environments. I don't know about you, but I have absolutely no nostalgia for the bad old days. If there are newer, better ways to do things, we'd be fools not to give them a try.

OK, back to power naps. The strategy that underlies this concept, for many people, is that they take place sometime between the time when our work related responsibilities for the day begin and the time when they end. In other words, almost any time during your workday is (potentially) fair game. That allows the power napper to be quite judicious in selecting the optimum time for the nap itself. But what about those who don't have jobs outside the home? Don't worry. Power naps are for you too. Homemakers, people running home-based businesses, and virtually anyone in a situation that can benefit from a recharge can benefit from a power nap. Many have found it an ideal way to meet the challenges of their day.

One of the amazing things about power napping is the level of dedication to be found amongst its devotees. It's the best evidence to me that it must really work. Most of them will swear that it plays in key role in their effectiveness, both on the job and in other aspects of life as well. Power nappers tend to have Type A personalities and are very task oriented. They use their naps to achieve their goals through rejuvenation, not simply for the pure pleasure associated with drifting off to a softer, gentler consciousness. That's where the "power" part of a power nap comes in. Some people take vitamins to give them energy. People who take power naps sleep their way to success. (OK, poor choice of words, if you have a dirty mind you might construe a different meaning...but I think you catch my drift.) Seriously, though, the power nappers I have met tell me that they have become quite proficient at quickly achieving their napping state and wake feeling both intellectually and physically refreshed and more prepared to get back to task.

Another creative form of napping is known as the preemptive nap. We can take these kinds of naps when we know we may have to postpone the start of our normal, nocturnal sleep and we want to offset the feelings of fatigue that usually accompanies that postponement. By taking a preemptive nap, we can go longer than usual and still maintain our emotional and physical balance. There is no consensus of opinion about this, however. In fact, there is dispute among sleep experts relative to the possibility of "banking" the restorative qualities of sleep. Nonetheless, field research reveals that many people are successful at working second jobs, pursuing after work educations, and simply getting more out of their lives by incorporating preemptive naps into their life schedules. While some folks have fully integrated preemptive napping into their life-style, most preemptive nappers use them more on an "as needed" basis.

Assuming this approach is a sensible one for you, let's get to the big question people inevitably ask. How long is a preemptive nap? Based on my totally non-scientific but doggedly ongoing survey of nappers, I would say that they vary anywhere from a thirty minute nap up to a little over an hour. Many of the people I have talked with tell me that for them a thirty minute nap seems the equivalent of a couple hours of nocturnal sleep in terms of restored energy and the ability to keep moving forward with their schedules. Even if you are not a scientific type, I think a little experimenting with nap lengths will put you in a good position to know how long your preemptive naps need to be. With the information gained from your personal napping experiment, you can develop a napping plan to meet most contingencies.

Another common nap type is the restorative nap. Just as the name implies, restorative naps can be used to sort of recharge ourselves when we have overextended or, more commonly, had an abbreviation of our normal nocturnal sleep. Think back to the last time you had to get up a couple of hours earlier than usual. Maybe you had to take someone to the airport for an early morning flight or possibly there was a work project that could only be scheduled before the rest of the staff reported for duty. Obviously there are dozens of reasons why our nocturnal sleep may be abbreviated. Just as obviously, when it is, we can count on hitting a wall of fatigue sometime later in the day. Restorative nap to the rescue. Fifteen minutes to a half hour will get your motor running and you will be right back on track.

Power naps, preemptive naps, and restorative naps all have their place. Some people benefit tremendously from each of these. But – call me old-fashioned -- my favorite nap type is still the good old reliable Pure Pleasure Nap. Now you may have a different name for it, but if you are a napper you know exactly what it is that I'm referring to. Right! It is the one that you take for the pure and simple joy that only a nap can provide. You don't take a Pure Pleasure Nap so you can work harder, longer and more effectively. You don't take it because you are going to have to stay up later in the evening and want to be sure you are alert and capable of high level functioning while postponing your normal nocturnal sleep onset. And though you may be a little tired, you are not taking it to make up for lost sleep. Nope. These reasons pale in comparison to your true motive. You take a Pure Pleasure Nap to elicit that incredibly freeing feeling that you only experience when you give yourself permission to just drift off, leaving behind the cares and stresses of everyday life.

Ahh....The Pure Pleasure Nap. There are few things in life that come close to its splendor. Yes, all naps are a gift, no question about that. But a Pure Pleasure Nap is that special gift that is wrapped in a way that promises the highest quality and most satisfying of all guilty pleasures. Even as I write this I am tempted to bolt to my couch and indulge myself. Sorry. As I was saying, this particular nap has everything going for it (and for you). It is not related to anything but itself. It is a stand-alone experience that shares company with any and all premier sensual experience you have ever had. It is not the symphony, but it is a symphony. It is not your favorite meal served in your favorite restaurant, but again it is. It is not the ocean breeze pushing your hair away as you face a sunset from the bow of a luxury liner, but actually it is. Well, you get the picture. I don't call it a Pure Pleasure Nap for no reason. The possibilities are as boundless as your own limitless imagination.

Now for the difficult part. How long should it be? Well, remember the ice cream and the pizza pie? Yes, even a Pure Pleasure Nap, alas, has some limitations (in terms of quantity – definitely not of quality!). I'll make this quick.

I probably should have mentioned in the A Little Science Goes A Long Ways chapter. Sorry. Anyway, our science friends have discovered that sleep occurs in five stages.

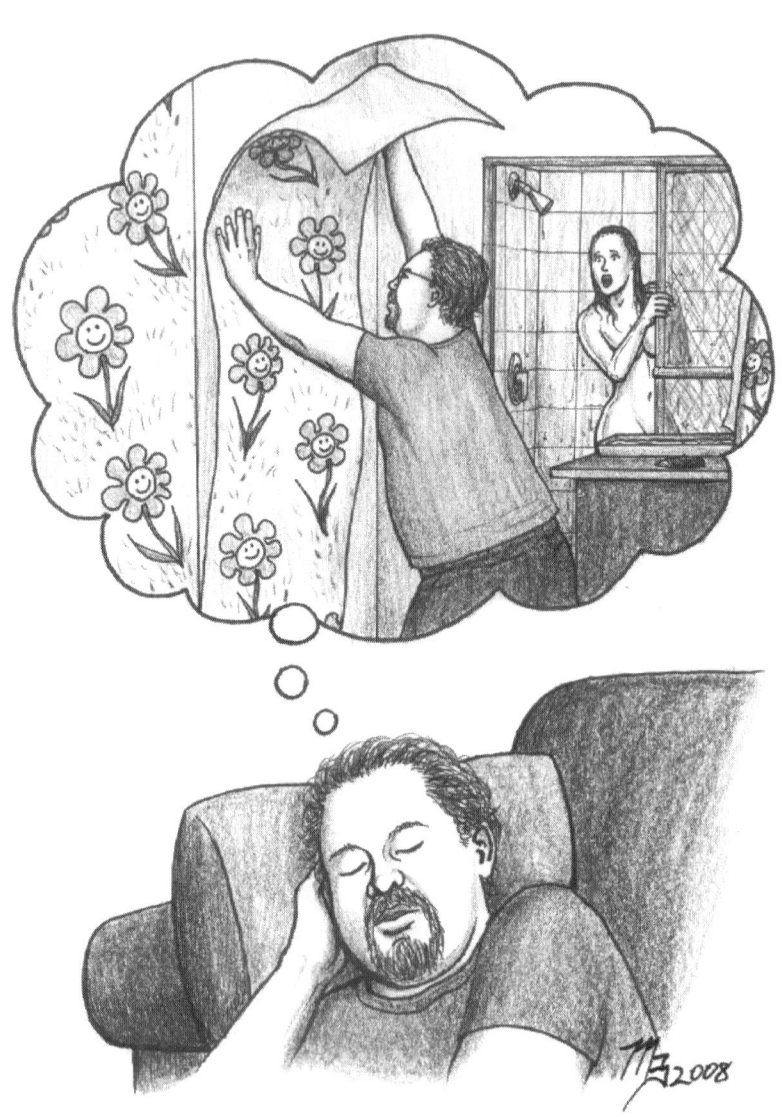

Each stage is characterized by a specific brain wave pattern and each stage of sleep has a particular quality. You will be refreshed and renewed in many ways by napping through the first three or four of these stages. The fifth stage is called the REM stage (stands for rapid eye movement, not the rock group). Although during nocturnal sleep you will cycle through the five stages maybe five or six times, you will enter the REM stage after about 90 initial minutes of sleep. It is arguable, but I recommend that you schedule your Pure Pleasure Nap in a way that avoids the onset of the REM cycle. Why? Well, first of all the brain wave activity during REM sleep most closely resembles that of a person who is fully awake and active. Who needs that when they are napping? Secondly, REM sleep is the cycle most associated with dreaming. Now, I enjoy a good dream as well as the next person. But, as I said I, enjoy a *good* dream. Unfortunately, like many other people I occasionally get stuck with that dream that involves me wall papering my neighbor's bathroom or finally cleaning out my cluttered garage. Nobody needs that kind of intrusion on their Pure Pleasure Nap. No one – trust me. So, my suggestion is to keep your nap to under two hours. You can always have your wallpaper or garage cleaning dream at night!

CHAPTER EIGHT

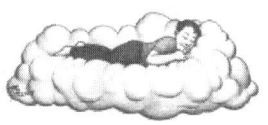

Speed Bumps Along
The Road To Nap Land

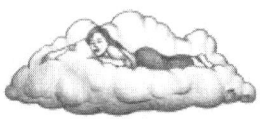

One of my more pessimistic friends has a tag line that he uses every time things don't work out perfectly or somehow fall short of his expectations. Usually with a shrug, he says, "Hey, nothing's easy." I don't think he is 100% correct, but he does have something of a point. Most things worthwhile aren't necessarily easy to obtain, but I think that there is another more universally accepted expression that is much more optimistic and serves all of us better. That expression is, "Practice makes perfect." If you were to carefully consider all of the things that you do during your day-to-day living, you might be surprised how many pretty complex activities just seem to come naturally – they don't seem to require any special attention at all. But here's my point – at one time, before you mastered these activities, they did require your close attention, focused concentration, and there is a pretty good chance that even then you may have failed a couple of times before you "got it right". Napping, for many of us, just seems to come naturally. After all, most of us had plenty of practice when we were very, very young! Of course most of us also learned how to walk at a very early age and still manage to occasionally trip over our own feet. And in all probability you were talking a blue streak by the time you were three years old and still occasionally get "tongue tied" or can't seem to pull up that one word that makes you sentence intelligible. Napping can be the exact same way. There are any number of reasons why, despite our best laid plan, that we are not able to drift off to nap land. To help, I have listed some of the major "failure to launch" scenarios and possible remedies that can be incorporated into your napping strategies.

It is an interesting paradox. One of the most common reasons given for napping is to reduce stress or compensate for the effects of stress. It makes sense; stress takes both an emotional and a physical toll on us. While naps are not a long-term solution to stress management, they can provide our bodies an opportunity to give up some of the physical tension associated with stress (you know, the stiff neck, sore back, general muscle tightness) and also the opportunity to take a brief respite from the environment that may be contributing to our stress. The paradox is that often it is the very stress symptoms that we are attempting to alleviate that prevent us from drifting off and gaining the benefits promised by a short nap. There are many ways to skirt past moderate levels of stress and get on to your "therapeutic" nap.

If you have experienced some difficulty moving your nap forward, my first suggestion is that you prepare yourself as you would for any nap; optimal location selected, napping time-frame established, any necessary accouterments in place. Now, add about five minutes to your napping schedule. This is the time that you are going to use to more fully prepare yourself for nap "lift off". Settle in, adjust your body so you are comfortable. Now, take two or three nice deep, even breaths and with your eyes closed, say to yourself, *"I am breathing in relaxation"* (as you breath in) and *"I am breathing out tension"* (yep, as you exhale). You can continue this simple mantra for several breaths and in many cases it will be all you need to get yourself on the way to nap land. What is happening is really very simple: you are giving yourself a wholly attainable self-suggestion (let's face it, those *are* our favorite kind of suggestion, aren't they?) and at the same time you are taking your mind away from what may be most immediately distracting you from a nap enhancing sense of relaxation. Don't be concerned that this strategy seems too simple – it works for most of us, most of the time.

There is another speed bump that nappers sometimes encounter. It has to do with timing. We have already established that anytime is a good time for a nap, but that may not always prove to be exactly true for you. It may be that another time is a better time for you. What do I mean? Well, it seems to always be easier to nap when we are actually feeling tired, but sometimes, say in the case of a preemptive nap, we aren't tired at all. Ever try to put the square peg into the round hole? It can be done, of course, but neither the peg nor the hole are ever quite the same afterwards! The lesson here is not to force the issue. Sure, give it a try. And if you are not successful – no big deal, give it another try a little later. But remember, frustration almost never leads to success in napping. Don't try to "force" your nap, like so many other things in life, coaxing is always going to be more effective. If you experience some napping resistance, you will almost always be better off to back off your napping attempt and try a little later on. Before you make your next attempt, ask yourself if you know why you didn't drift off the last time. Were you too tense (read previous paragraph, please)? Did you really have the time to take the nap? Were the environmental conditions (noise, temperature, people around you) just too nap inhibiting? Remember, "Practice makes perfect", and you may have to practice napping in some less than perfectly nap-friendly environments to get your napping "legs". Once you've got them, you will be able to nap at the drop of a hat just about anywhere you chose.

I have made a point of distinguishing between naps and regular nocturnal sleep. And with good reason; they are much different from both a physiological perspective and a social perspective. They do, however, have some characteristics in common. When it comes to difficulty in achieving a napping state, I suggest that you consider what past difficulties you may have encountered with your regular nocturnal sleep and, more importantly, how you overcame them. I'm not referring to certified insomnia, just the occasional inability to easily fall asleep. It happens to all of us, gratefully, not too often. Common reasons include basic over-tiredness, digestive interference (think late night pizza), racing mind syndrome (omigosh! I have tons to do tomorrow), aches and pains (my lawn is raked and my back is killing me!). When nocturnal sleep eludes us, sometimes a warm glass of milk or reading a book will trip us into slumber. With a reluctant nap, that type of alternative just isn't practical. What we can do, though, is move our minds away from the "here and now"

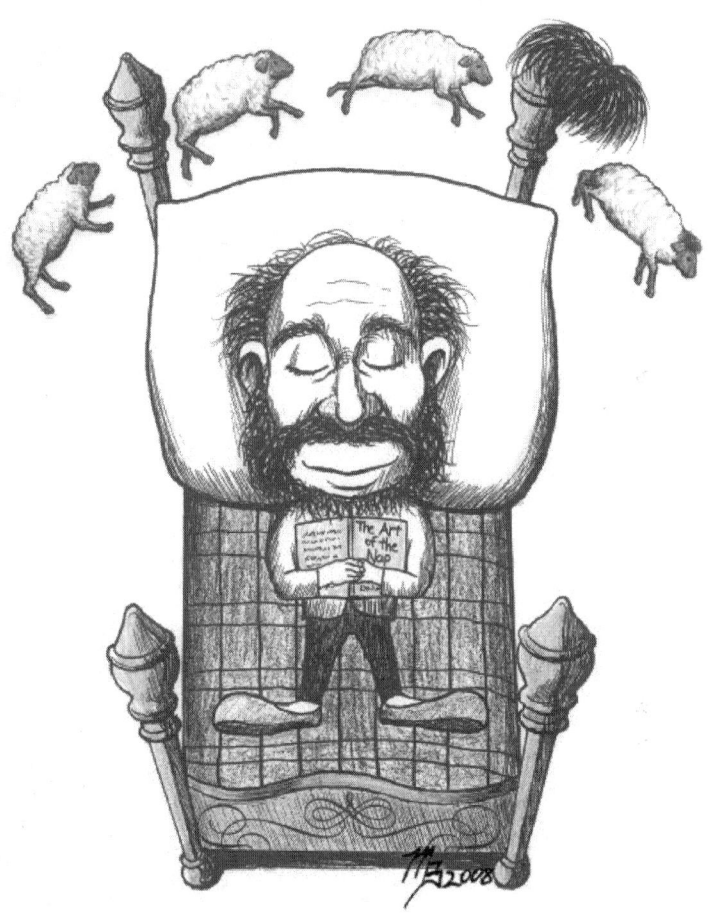

just a bit by…ready for this? Counting sheep. Umm. I can almost hear you now. Counting sheep! Are you kidding, that only works in cartoons and comic books! Well, actually it works quite well. If you have the creative imagination that allows you to conjure a series of laconic sheep slowly leaping over a fence as you count them off; one, two, three, four, five (you get the picture), give it a try. I believe you will be very pleasantly surprised how effective it can be. If the idea of inviting a flock (or is it a bevy?) of conjured sheep into your personal nap space leaves you a little cold, try this. Instead of counting sheep, count cows – no, I'm just kidding here. What I would like to suggest is that you do a simple backwards count to yourself to help clear your mind of nap distracting thoughts and to distract your mind from your immediate physical issues (soreness, tummy ache, and the specter of a too busy tomorrow). With your eyes closed, begin your count at 100 and count slowly towards zero. I'm guessing you won't make it to 50 before you have drifted off to your much deserved and earned nap.

This last speed bump is a little different from the others mentioned. It has to do with the people in your life. Specifically, those that you nap around. You might remember that in the Foreword of The Art of The Nap (yeah, yeah, I know – who reads the Foreword?) a distinction was made between those of us that value and take naps and those that consider them to be a complete waste of time. This is a pretty large breech in attitudes and behaviors and can pose some problems – mostly, it seems, for the nappers. If you live or work around napping naysayers, save your breath on trying to convince them of the virtues of napping. But you are way within your rights to let them know that you respect their opinion and in turn expect the same respect from them. For optimum reception I suggest a smile in your voice when you communicate this (best to save the snarl for another time – ah, the power of a little honey). I don't believe it is the role of we nappers to proselytize napping to others, but I know one napper who made a short list of benefits that accrue not only to the napper but to those around the napper. She has been known to hand this list, printed on a three by five card, to folks who question her napping ways. This is a really smart woman, her list has three benefits for the napper and five for the people or organization around the napper. Want her list? Sorry, but the teacher in me knows that the list you develop yourself will be the one that serves you best. Think about it.

I hope these simple suggestions help in the few instances when a nap may be eluding you. Do try them if the occasion presents itself and, not to be boorish about it, please remember that practice does make perfect.

CHAPTER NINE

Time to….Nap!

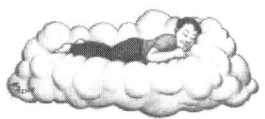
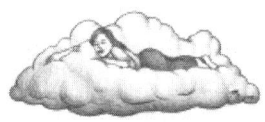

It's amazing how time flies when you're having fun, but we've actually now reached the final chapter of The Art of The Nap. Have you ever noticed when listening to a really good lecture or speech, that no matter how interesting the subject or captivating the speaker, the most dreaded phrase is *"…in summary"?* This is usually the signal that the person delivering the message is about to deliver it all over again, albeit in a somewhat condensed format! Egads! No worry, I won't do that to you.

After all that napping ground that we have covered to this point, I realize that it may seem like a most peculiar place to ask the question, "What is the chief benefit of napping?" After all, wouldn't that question fit more comfortably near the beginning of the book rather than at the end? In all fairness, I guess the answer could be "Yes." And I know that in a somewhat global way the restorative features of napping as well as the overall pleasantness of the napping have been cited. But I remind you that in the Foreword I dedicated this book to nappers – not napper wannabes. The intent was to validate, celebrate, and enhance the napping experience of my fellow nappers, not to "sell" the concept of napping to those that are skeptical or outright anti-napping. I will leave the apologetics and proselytizing to others. The very thought of that crusader role leaves me drained and heading for the nearest napping nest I can find. I much prefer preaching to the choir, reaching out to my fellow napping enthusiasts throughout the world.

It should be clear by this point that the benefits of regular napping are clearly too numerous to count. I hope that The Art of The Nap has unveiled some of the nearly infinite ways that naps can be used to enhance your energy, stamina and productivity, and has suggested some useful measures which will lead you to better, even more satisfying naps. I certainly hope that I conveyed the concept that naps can and should be incorporated into your lifestyle not simply for pragmatic purposes, but for the sheer joy and pleasure that they provide as well. If you missed this last concept or it didn't seem emphasized strongly enough, let me say it one last time. If you remember nothing else from this book, never forget the following dictum: *a nap, taken for any reason whatsoever, is still a nap. It is a wonderful pleasure that we can give our selves that has absolutely no down side at all; there are no calories involved, it is not habit forming, it won't elevate your cholesterol count, and a nap will never, ever leave you with a hangover.* There is also no "napping tax" and although I'm not an attorney, I'm confident that they are still legal in all 50 states (and in most foreign nations too, presumably).

I once heard someone refer to her naps being "guilty pleasures", in the same way that some people think of chocolate or rich desserts. No, no, no! Quite the contrary, naps are just plain and simple – all good. But you are a napper, you already know this. Nap away – no guilt! Unlike fattening foods, napping won't harm your health. To the contrary, your body will reap enormous benefits from being so well rested.

Have you heard the expression, "leave good enough alone"? For me, if I can wake refreshed, relaxed and invigorated from my nap, I am prepared to declare victory. Improving my mental outlook (uh…I guess that would be *mood*), sharpening my attention to detail and being ready for more action are incredible dividends for a thirty minute nap investment. It seems that is not good enough for all nappers, though. And who am I to argue. Each of us becomes expert in our naps and some feel confident in recommending benefits that are far out of my personal experience. Take a cruise through the Internet and be prepared to be amazed at the claims that are made for the simple nap. Some claim to have lost weight through napping (I guess you can't eat while your taking your nap), others make fairly sweeping statements concerning various health benefits associated with napping. And trust me, I am not impugning the validity of their statements and certainly not their sincerity. I just don't have the time necessary to closely examine the methodology of research (to say nothing of the requisite expertise) used to arrive at these conclusions. There's really no need to, as I am more than content with what I get from my naps. I hope you are too. Happy napping, friend. It's time for mine right now!

REFERENCES

INFORMATION ON SLEEP CYCLES

Psychology, Themes and Variations (7th Edition)
Wayne Weiten, Thomson Wadsworth

DISASTERS ASSOCIATED WITH SLEEP DEPRIVATION

http://www.guardian.co.uk/uk/2000/jul/09/anthonybrowne.
the observer1

http://www.timeshighereducation.co.uk/story.asp?storyCod
e=151939&sectioncode=26

http://space.about.com/b/2006/06/19/sleep-deprivation-
and-the-challenger-disaster.htm

INSOMNIA

http://www.emedicinehealth.com/insomnia/article_em.htm

SCIENCE OF SLEEP

http://www.bbc.co.uk/science/humanbody/sleep/articles/
whatissleep.shtml

Printed in Great Britain
by Amazon

34992676R00037